THROMBOPHILIA

UNDERSTANDING EVERYTHING ABOUT THROMBOPHILIA

DR. KATE .P

Contents

CHAPTER ONE 3

INTRODUCTION..3

Symptoms 4

When to visit a physician 5

Reasons 6

RISK ELEMENTS 7

COMMITMENTS 9

Getting Ready for Your Consultation 12

What you're capable of...13

CHAPTER TWO 14

Prepare a list of inquiries for your physician...........14

What to anticipate from your physician 17

What you can accomplish in the interim 18

Exams and diagnosis 19

MEDICATIONS AND SUBTLES 21

WAY OF LIFE AND DOMESTIC MEDICINE 25

THE END 28

CHAPTER ONE

INTRODUCTION

When a blood clot stops one or more of your veins, usually in your legs, you get thrombophilia (throm-boe-fluh-BY-tis). Thrombophlebitis, often known as phlebitis, is a rare condition that can damage the veins in your neck or arms.

The afflicted vein may be deep within a muscle, resulting in deep vein thrombosis (DVT), or it may be close to the skin's surface, causing superficial thrombophlebitis. A lengthy period of inactivity, trauma, or surgery can all result in thrombophilia. Individuals with varicose veins may develop superficial thrombophlebitis.

Your risk of developing major health issues, such as a pulmonary embolism a blockage of an artery in your lungs is increased when you have a clot in a deep vein. Medication to thin the blood is typically used to treat deep vein thrombosis. Sometimes blood thinners are used to treat superficial thrombophlebitis as well.

Symptoms

Symptoms of superficial thrombophlebitis include:

Pain, warmth, and soreness in the afflicted area

Swelling and redness

Symptoms of deep vein thrombosis include:

Anguish

Bloating

You could see a red, tough, and sensitive cord just beneath the skin's surface when a vein near the surface becomes infected. A leg's deep vein might become inflamed, sore, and painful when this happens.

When to visit a physician

If you have a red, swollen, or sore vein, you should see your doctor very once, especially if you have one or more thrombophlebitis risk factors. See an emergency hospital if you experience discomfort and swelling in your legs, as well as shortness of breath or chest pain that hurts when you take deep breaths. These symptoms could be indicative of deep vein thrombosis, which raises the possibility that a blood clot may become dislodged and pass through your veins and into your lungs.

Reasons

A blood clot is the cause of thrombophlebitis. Blood clots can result from a variety of factors, primarily anything that impairs blood circulation. A blood clot that results in thrombophlebitis may be brought on by:

A vein injury

An hereditary disease of blood coagulation

being immobilized for extended periods of time, as when admitted to the hospital

RISK ELEMENTS

There is an increased risk of thrombophlebitis if you:

Are bedridden for an extended period of time, following surgery, a heart attack, or an injury, like fracturing a leg

Have you experienced a stroke that left your arms or legs immobile?

implant a catheter a thin, flexible tube in a central vein for the purpose of treating a medical condition that could irritate the blood vessel wall and reduce blood flow.

Are you expecting or just gave birth, which could indicate that the veins in your legs and pelvis are under more pressure?

Use hormone replacement treatment or birth control tablets, as these may increase the risk of blood clotting.

possess an inclination to form blood clots readily or a family history of a blood-clotting illness

are still for extended periods of time, like while seated in an automobile or an aircraft

are more than 60 years old

Possess varicose veins, a typical cause of thrombophlebitis superficial

Your risk of thrombophlebitis increases with the number of risk factors you have. Before engaging in prolonged periods of inactivity, such as following an elective operation or during a lengthy flight or vehicle ride, make sure to discuss preventive actions with your doctor if you have one or more risk factors.

COMMITMENTS

Complications are uncommon when thrombophlebitis occurs in a superficial vein, which is located just beneath the surface. On the other hand, deep vein thrombosis, a dangerous medical disease, could develop if the clot happens in a deep vein. There is a higher chance of major consequences if it occurs. Possible complications include:

embolism in the lung. A dislodged portion of a deep vein clot has the potential to go to your lungs and create an embolism, which is an artery blockage that could be fatal.

phlebetic syndrome after. Post-thrombotic syndrome, another name for this illness, can appear months or even years after deep vein thrombosis. In the affected leg, post-phlebetic syndrome can result in persistent discomfort, swelling, and a heaviness that may be incapacitating. Deep vein thrombosis can be prevented or treated by compression stockings worn for at least two years from the onset of the disorder.

The vein valves in your legs may potentially sustain damage from deep vein thrombosis. The valves in veins stop blood from flowing backwards as it is progressively forced upwards toward your heart. A malfunctioning valve in the veins of your legs can lead to a number of issues:

veins that are variable. Varicose veins can develop from your veins ballooning due to blood pooling.

Growing. Sometimes the pooling might get so excessive that it causes edema, or swelling in the legs.

Discoloration of the skin. Discoloration may happen as a result of persistent swelling and increased strain on your skin. Skin sores can occasionally appear. Give your doctor a call if you think a skin ulcer is developing.

Getting Ready for Your Consultation

See your doctor as soon as possible if you experience any thrombophlebitis symptoms, such as a red, swollen, or sore vein. Call 911 or your local emergency number if the vein swelling and pain are severe, or if you have any other symptoms (such as shortness of breath or blood in your cough) that could point to a blood clot in your lungs.

Here are some resources to help you prepare for your appointment and know what to anticipate from your doctor, if you have time before it.

What you're capable of

Jot down any symptoms you're having, even if they don't seem to be connected to thrombophlebitis.

Important personal information should be noted, particularly if there is a family history of blood-clotting issues or if you have lately engaged in prolonged periods of inactivity, such as air travel. Additionally, let your doctor know about your travel itinerary if you intend to travel and are worried about your risk of thrombophlebitis.

Enumerate any drug you take, along with any vitamins and supplements.

CHAPTER TWO

If at all feasible, have someone drive you to the hospital or emergency room. You might find it challenging to operate a vehicle, so it's beneficial to have a support person accompany you to your visit to ensure you remember everything your doctor says. Give yourself immediate medical attention by dialing 911 or your local emergency number if you experience signs of a pulmonary embolism, such as shortness of breath or chest pain.

Prepare a list of inquiries for your physician

Since you don't have much time with your doctor, being prepared with a list of questions will help you get the most out of your visit. In the event that time runs out, prioritize your list of questions from most to least important. Basic inquiries for your doctor regarding thrombophlebitis include:

What is probably the root of my illness?

What other factors could be causing my symptoms?

Which tests will I require?

Which of the available treatments would you suggest?

What kind of exercise is suitable for me now that I have a thrombophlebitis diagnosis? What happens once my clot disappears?

What are the alternatives you propose to the main strategy?

I also suffer from various medical issues. How can I and my partner best manage these conditions?

Do I have to abide by any dietary restrictions?

Is there a generic version of the medication you are recommending?

What adverse effects should I anticipate from this medication?

Are there any printed materials, such as brochures, available for me to take home? Which websites would you advise people to visit?

You'll probably be asked a lot of questions by your doctor. Being prepared to respond to them could buy you extra time to discuss any topics you'd like to cover in greater detail. Your physician might inquire:

When did you start feeling the effects?

Do you constantly experience symptoms, or do they come and go?

What level of severity do you have?

What further health issues do you have?

In the previous three months, have you undergone any significant injuries or surgeries?

Have you miscarried during a pregnancy before?

Which medications do you take at the moment?

What appears to make your symptoms better or worse, if anything?

Do you have a family history of blood clot-related health issues?

What you can accomplish in the interim

You can start certain self-care practices prior to your doctor's appointment. To ease any discomfort, elevate the leg that is afflicted and apply a warm washcloth as a compress on the affected area. Make sure your doctor knows if you choose to take an ibuprofen (Advil, Motrin IB, and other brands). Drugs may interfere with other blood clot-dissolving drugs that your physician prescribes.

Exams and diagnosis

Your doctor will first ask you about any discomfort you've experienced before checking for any damaged veins close to the skin's surface to make the diagnosis of thrombophlebitis. Your doctor may order one of the following tests to identify if you have deep vein thrombosis or superficial thrombophlebitis:

blood examination. A naturally occurring chemical called D dimer dissolves blood clots, and almost everyone who has a blood clot has elevated blood levels of this substance. D dimer levels, however, can also be raised under different circumstances. Therefore, a D dimer test may point to the need for more testing but is not definitive. It is also helpful in ruling out deep vein thrombosis and identifying individuals who are at risk of recurrent thrombophlebitis.

ultrasonic. Sound waves are injected into your leg by a transducer, which resembles a wand and is moved over the injured area. Sound waves enter your leg tissue, bounce back, and are then converted by a computer into a moving picture that appears on a video screen. There might be a clot in the picture.

CT scan. A computed tomography (CT) scan may reveal whether a clot is present and offer visual images of your lungs.

MEDICATIONS AND SUBTLES

Your doctor could advise self-care measures such as heating the painful area, elevating the affected leg, and taking an over-the-counter nonsteroidal anti-inflammatory medicine (NSAID) if thrombophlebitis develops in a vein close beneath the skin. In most cases, there is no need for hospitalization, and the situation gets much better in about a month.

Additionally, your physician can suggest one of the following therapies for thrombophlebitis, such as deep vein thrombosis:

drugs that thin the blood. An injection of a blood-thinning (anticoagulant) drug, such as fondaparinux (Arixtra) or low molecular weight heparin, will stop clots from growing if you have deep vein thrombosis. Following the first course of treatment, using the oral anticoagulant warfarin (Coumadin) for a few months keeps clots from getting bigger. If your physician prescribes warfarin, carefully follow the recommendations on how to take the prescription. Excessive bleeding is one of the most dangerous side effects of warfarin. Taken orally, rivaroxaban (Xarelto) is a more recent blood thinner that may have a lower bleeding risk.

drugs that dissolve clots. Thrombolysis is the term for this kind of therapy. These drugs, which break up blood clots, such alteplase (Activase), are used to treat deep vein thrombosis that is severe or in some circumstances if the condition also involves a pulmonary embolus (blood clot in the lung).

Stockings with compression. Compression stockings with prescription strength assist lower the risk of deep vein thrombosis complications and stop swelling from returning. It's possible that your doctor will advise you to wear these for at least two years.

Sort through. A filter may occasionally be placed into the vena cava, the major vein in your abdomen, to stop blood clots that break loose in leg veins from getting into your lungs. This is particularly common if you are unable to take blood thinners. When the filter is no longer required, it is usually removed. Consult your doctor about whether and when to get a filter removed if you have one installed.

stripping varicose veins. Varicose vein stripping is a surgical technique that your doctor might perform to remove varicose veins that are painful or cause recurrent thrombophlebitis. During this treatment, tiny incisions are made to remove a lengthy vein. Because deeper veins in the leg handle the greater blood volumes, vein removal won't disrupt circulation in your leg. Cosmetic reasons are another motivation to have this operation done. Your doctor could advise you to wear compression stockings in addition to vein stripping.

WAY OF LIFE AND DOMESTIC MEDICINE

Ankles and calves that swell from sitting might result after extended flights or vehicle rides. Additionally, the inactivity raises your risk of developing thrombophlebitis in your leg veins. In an effort to stop a blood clot from forming:

Go for a stroll. Take a once-hour or so stroll around the cabin of the aircraft if you're flying. Every hour or so, if you're driving, pull over and take a stroll.

If you have to remain seated, alternate between your legs. At least ten times each hour, flex your ankles or gently press your feet against the ground or footrest in front of you.

To lower your risk of deep vein thrombosis, take the following extra precautions when traveling by automobile or during flights that run more than four hours:

Steer clear of tight apparel.

To prevent dehydration, consume a lot of nonalcoholic beverages.

At least once each hour, go for a walk to stretch your calves.

Speak with your doctor before to your flight if you have a higher risk of deep vein thrombosis. He or she might advise you to make use of:

Stockings with compression

any blood-thinning drug that is prescribed and taken as directed

THE END